MW01285348

6 Full-Length SBAC Grade 3 Math Practice Tests

Extra Test Prep to Help Ace the SBAC Grade 3 Math Test

By

Michael Smith & Reza Nazari

6 Full-Length SBAC Grade 3 Math Practice Tests

Published in the United State of America By

The Math Notion

Web: WWW.MathNotion.Com

Email: info@Mathnotion.com

About the Author

Michael Smith has been a math instructor for over a decade now. He holds a master's degree in Management. Since 2006, Michael has devoted his time to both teaching and developing exceptional math learning materials. As a Math instructor and test prep expert, Michael has worked with thousands of students. He has used the feedback of his students to develop a unique study program that can be used by students to drastically improve their math score fast and effectively.

- **SAT Math Practice Book**
- **ACT Math Practice Book**
- **GRE Math Practice Book**
- **Common Core Math Practice Book**
- **many Math Education Workbooks, Exercise Books and Study Guides**

As an experienced Math teacher, Mr. Smith employs a variety of formats to help students achieve their goals: He tutors online and in person, he teaches students in large groups, and he provides training materials and textbooks through his website and through Amazon.

You can contact Michael via email at:

info@Mathnotion.com

Prepare for the SBAC Grade 3 Math test with a perfect practice book!

The surest way to practice your SBAC Math test-taking skills is with simulated exams. This comprehensive practice book with 6 full length and realistic SBAC Math practice tests help you measure your exam readiness, find your weak areas, and succeed on the SBAC Math test. The detailed answers and explanations for each SBAC Math question help you master every aspect of the SBAC Math.

6 Full-length SBAC Grade 3 Math Practice Tests is a prestigious resource to help you succeed on the SBAC Math test. This perfect practice book features:

- Content 100% aligned with the SBAC test
- Six full-length SBAC Math practice tests similar to the actual test in length, format, question types, and degree of difficulty
- Detailed answers and explanations for the SBAC Math practice questions
- Written by SBAC Math top instructors and experts

After completing this hands-on exercise book, you will gain confidence, strong foundation, and adequate practice to succeed on the SBAC Math test.

WWW.MathNotion.COM

… So Much More Online!

✓ FREE Math Lessons

✓ More Math Learning Books!

✓ Mathematics Worksheets

✓ Online Math Tutors

For a PDF Version of This Book

Please Visit WWW.MathNotion.com

Contents

SBAC Math Practice Tests

Smarter Balanced Assessment Consortium (SBAC) test assesses student mastery of the common core State Standards.

The SBAC is a computer adaptive test. It means that there is a set of test questions in a variety of question types that adjust to each student based on the student's answers to previous questions. This section includes a range of items types, such as selecting several correct responses for one item, typing out a response, fill--in short answers/tables, graphing, drag and drop, etc.

On computer adaptive tests, if the correct answer is chosen, the next question will be harder. If the answer given is incorrect, the next question will be easier. This also means that once an answer is selected on the computer it cannot be changed.

In this section, there are 2 complete SBAC Math Tests that reflect the format and question types on SBAC. On a real SBAC Math test, the number of questions varies and there are about 30 questions.

Let your student take these tests to see what score he or she will be able to receive on a real SBAC test.

Time to Test

Time to refine your skill with a practice examination

Take a REAL SBAC Mathematics test to simulate the test day experience. After you've finished, score your test using the answer key.

Before You Start

- You'll need a pencil and scratch papers to take the test.
- For this practice test, don't time yourself. Spend time as much as you need.
- It's okay to guess. You won't lose any points if you're wrong.
- After you've finished the test, review the answer key to see where you went wrong.

Calculators are not permitted for Grade 3 SBAC Tests

Good Luck!

SBAC GRADE 3 MAHEMATICS REFRENCE MATERIALS

LENGTH

Customary	Metric
1 mile (mi) = 1,760 yards (yd)	1 kilometer (km) = 1,000 meters (m)
1 yard (yd) = 3 feet (ft)	1 meter (m) = 100 centimeters (cm)
1 foot (ft) = 12 inches (in.)	1 centimeter (cm) = 10 millimeters (mm)

VOLUME AND CAPACITY

Customary	Metric
1 gallon (gal) = 4 quarts (qt)	1 liter (L) = 1,000 milliliters (mL)
1 quart (qt) = 2 pints (pt.)	
1 pint (pt.) = 2 cups (c)	
1 cup (c) = 8 fluid ounces (Fl oz)	

WEIGHT AND MASS

Customary	Metric
1 ton (T) = 2,000 pounds (lb.)	1 kilogram (kg) = 1,000 grams (g)
1 pound (lb.) = 16 ounces (oz)	1 gram (g) = 1,000 milligrams (mg)

Time

1 year = 12 months

1 year = 52 weeks

1 week = 7 days

1 day = 24 hours

1 hour = 60 minutes

1 minute = 60 seconds

Smarter Balanced Assessment Consortium (SBAC)

SBAC Practice Test 1

Mathematics

GRADE 3

❖ **30 questions**

❖ **There is no time limit for this practice test.**

❖ **Calculators are NOT permitted for this practice test**

Administered Month Year

1) Olivia has 93 pastilles. She wants to put them in boxes of 3 pastilles. How many boxes does she need?

   A. 30

   B. 31

   C. 34

   D. 28

2) There are 82 students from Riddle Elementary school at the library on Tuesday. The other 64 students in the school are practicing in the classroom. Which number sentence shows the total number of students in Riddle Elementary school?

   A. $82 + 64$

   B. $82 - 64$

   C. 82×64

   D. $82 \div 64$

3) Martin earns There are 6 numbers in the box below. Which of the following list shows only odd numbers from the numbers in the box?

13, 30, 24, 18, 73, 39

   A. 13, 24, 18

   B. 13, 39, 73

   C. 13, 30, 24

   D. 24, 18, 30

4) Classroom A contains 7 rows of chairs with 5 chairs per row. If classroom B has three times as many chairs, which number sentence can be used to find the number of chairs in classroom B?

A. $7 \times 5 + 3$

B. $7 + 5 \times 3$

C. $7 \times 5 \times 3$

D. $7 + 5 + 3$

5) There are 2 days in a weekend. There are 24 hours in day. How many hours are in a weekend?

A. 48

B. 96

C. 168

D. 200

6) Emily described a number using these clues:

Three-digit odd numbers that have a 7 in the hundreds place and a 3 in the tens place. Which number could fit Ella's description?

A. 727

B. 737

C. 732

D. 736

7) A cafeteria menu had spaghetti with meatballs for $8 and bean soup for $7 How much would it cost to buy three plates of spaghetti with meatballs and three bowls of bean soup?

    A. 15

    B. 24

    C. 45

    D. 135

8) This clock shows a time after 12:00 PM. What time was it 1 hours and 45 minutes ago?

    A. 12:45 PM

    B. 1:45 PM

    C. 1: 15 PM

    D. 12:30 PM

9) A football team is buying new uniforms. Each uniform cost $30. The team wants to buy 12uniforms.

Which equation represents a way to find the total cost of the uniforms?

    A. $(30 \times 10) + (1 \times 12) = 300 + 12$

    B. $(30 \times 10) + (10 \times 1) = 300 + 10$

    C. $(30 \times 10) + (30 \times 2) = 300 + 60$

    D. $(12 \times 10) + (10 \times 20) = 120 + 200$

10) Mia's goal is to save $160 to purchase her favorite bike.

- In January, she saved $46.

- In February, she saved $38.

How much money does Mia need to save in March to be able to purchase her favorite bike?

A. $28

B. $30

C. $52

D. $76

11) Michelle has 84 old books. She plans to send all of them to the library in their area. If she puts the books in boxes which can hold 4 books, which of the following equations can be used to find the number of boxes she will use?

A. $84 + 4 = $ _____

B. $84 \times 4 = $ _____

C. $84 - 4 = $ _____

D. $84 \div 4 = $ _____

12) Which number is made up of 5 hundreds, 7 tens, and 6 ones?

A. 5076

B. 576

C. 567

D. 675

13) Elise had 956 cards. Then, she gave 352 of the cards to her friend Alice. After that, Elise lost 250 cards.

Which equation can be used to find the number of cards Elise has now?

A. $956 - 352 + 250 =$ _____

B. $956 - 352 - 250 =$ _____

C. $956 + 352 + 250 =$ _____

D. $956 + 352 - 250 =$ _____

14) The length of the following rectangle is 9 centimeters and its width is 4 centimeters. What is the area of the rectangle?

A. 12 cm^2

B. 21 cm^2

C. 36 cm^2

D. 22 cm^2

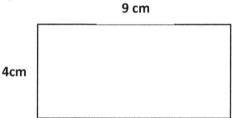

15) Look at the spinner above. On which color is the spinner most likely to land?

A. Red

B. Green

C. Yellow

D. None

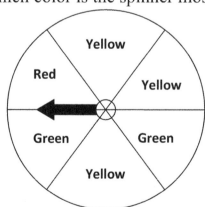

16) A group of third grade students recorded the following distances that they jumped.

23 inches	36 inches	24 inches	28 inches
36 inches	33 inches	25 inches	34 inches
32 inches	28 inches	34 inches	36 inches

What is the distance that was jumped most often?

A. 23

B. 24

C. 32

D. 36

17) Emma flew 3,391 miles from Los Angeles to New York City. What is the number of miles Emma flew rounded to the nearest thousand?

A. 2,000

B. 2,400

C. 2,500

D. 3,000

18) To what number is the arrow pointing?

A. 24

B. 28

C. 30

D. 32

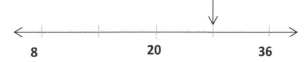

19) A number sentence such as $25 + Z = 92$ can be called an equation. If this equation is true, then which of the following equations is not true?

A. $92 - 25 = Z$

B. $92 - Z = 25$

C. $Z - 92 = 25$

D. $Z = 67$

20) Use the picture below to answer the question. Which fraction shows the shaded part of this square?

A. $\dfrac{87}{100}$

B. $\dfrac{87}{10}$

C. $\dfrac{87}{1,000}$

D. $\dfrac{8}{100}$

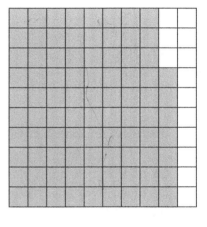

21) Which number correctly completes the number sentence $80 \times 35 =?$

A. 350

B. 900

C. 1,250

D. 2,800

22) Which number correctly completes the subtraction sentence

$7000 - 858 =$ _____ ?

A. 6,142

B. 7,452

C. 742

D. 7,458

23) Jason packs 12 boxes with flashcards. Each box holds 30 flashcards. How many flashcards Jason can pack into these boxes?

A. 86

B. 860

C. 530

D. 360

24) Which of the following statements describes the number 26,586?

A. The sum of two thousands, 6 thousands, five hundreds, eighty tens, and six ones

B. The sum of sixty thousands, 2 thousands, five hundreds, eight tens, and six ones

C. The sum of twenty thousands, 6 thousands, fifty hundreds, eighty tens, and six ones

D. The sum of twenty thousands, 6 thousands, five hundreds, eight tens, and six ones

25) The following models are the same size and each divided into equal parts.

The models can be used to write two fractions.

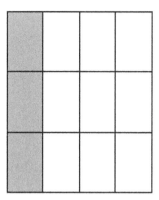 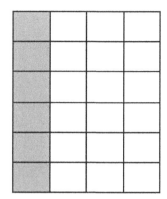

Based on the models, which of the following statements is true?

A. $\frac{3}{12}$ is bigger than $\frac{6}{24}$.

B. $\frac{3}{12}$ is smaller than $\frac{6}{24}$.

C. $\frac{3}{12}$ is equal to $\frac{6}{24}$.

D. We cannot compare these two fractions only by using the models.

26) What is the value of "A" in the following equation?

$$23 + A + 8 = 42$$

A. 10

B. 11

C. 14

D. 20

27) Emily has 144 stickers and she wants to give them to nine of her closest friends.

   If she gives them all an equal number of stickers, how many stickers will each

   of Emily's friends receive?

   A. 16

   B. 135

   C. 153

   D. 1,296

28) Use the models below to answer the question.

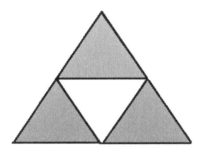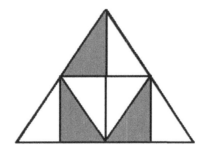

   Which statement about the models is true?

   A. Each shows the same fraction because they are the same size.

   B. Each shows a different fraction because they are different shapes.

   C. Each shows the same fraction because they both have 3 sections shaded.

   D. Each shows a different fraction because they both have 3 shaded sections but

   a different number of total sections.

29) Mr. smith usually eats TWO meals a day. How many meals does he eat in a week?

    A. 21

    B. 14

    C. 28

    D. 30

30) What is the value of A in the equation $56 \div A = 8$?

    A. 2

    B. 6

    C. 7

    D. 9

"This is the end of the practice test 1"

Smarter Balanced Assessment Consortium (SBAC)

SBAC Practice Test 2

Mathematics

GRADE 3

- ❖ **30 questions**
- ❖ **There is no time limit for this practice test.**
- ❖ **Calculators are NOT permitted for this practice test**

Administered Month Year

1) Mason is 15 months now and he usually eats four meals a day. How many meals does he eat in a week?

  A. 36

  B. 40

  C. 28

  D. 48

2) Which of the following list shows only fractions that are equivalent to $\frac{1}{3}$?

  A. $\frac{3}{9}, \frac{5}{15}, \frac{24}{72}$

  B. $\frac{6}{12}, \frac{5}{15}, \frac{9}{27}$

  C. $\frac{3}{9}, \frac{4}{15}, \frac{6}{18}$

  D. $\frac{3}{9}, \frac{5}{10}, \frac{8}{24}$

3) What mixed number is shown by the shaded rectangles?

  A. $2\frac{1}{3}$

  B. $2\frac{3}{4}$

  C. $3\frac{3}{4}$

  D. $2\frac{1}{4}$

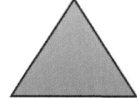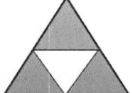

4) What number makes this equation true?

$$13 \times 5 = \square$$

A. 88

B. 65

C. 100

D. 108

5) Kayla has 120 red cards and 85 white cards. How many more red cards than white cards do Kayla have?

A. 17

B. 19

C. 35

D. 27

6) A number sentence is shown below.

$3 \times 5 \square 8 = 120$

What symbol goes into the box to make the number sentence true?

A. ×

B. ÷

C. +

D. −

7) Liam had 835 marbles. Then, he gave 432 of the cards to his friend Ethan. After

that, Liam lost 116 cards.

Which equation can be used to find the number of cards Eve has now?

A. 835 – 432 + 116 = ____

B. 835 – 432 – 116 = ____

C. 835 + 432 + 116 = ____

D. 835 + 432 – 116 = ____

8) What is the value of "B" in the following equation?

$$43 + B + 7 = 63$$

A. 16

B. 18

C. 22

D. 13

9) There are two different cards on the table.

- There are 3 rows that have 12 red cards in each row.

- There are 21 white cards.

How many cards are there on the table?

A. 25

B. 57

C. 33

D. 99

10) The perimeter of a square is 36units. Each side of this square is the same length.

What is the length of one side of the square in units?

A. 4

B. 5

C. 6

D. 8

11) Which of the following comparison of fractions is true?

A. $\frac{3}{5} = \frac{9}{15}$

B. $\frac{2}{5} > \frac{4}{10}$

C. $\frac{2}{5} < \frac{4}{10}$

D. $\frac{2}{5} < \frac{2}{10}$

12) The sum of 4 ten thousand, 7 hundred, and 8 tens can be expressed as what number in standard form?

A. 4,780

B. 40,780

C. 40,078

D. 40,708

13) One side of a square is 5 feet. What is the area of the square?

   A. 10

   B. 20

   C. 25

   D. 50

14) What is the perimeter of the following triangle?

   A. 28 inches

   B. 35 inches

   C. 48 inches

   D. 183 inches

12 inches   20 inches

16 inches

15) Moe has 460 cards. He wants to put them in boxes of 20 cards. How many boxes

   does he need?

   A. 20

   B. 21

   C. 22

   D. 23

16) There are 8 rows of chairs in a classroom with 7chairs in each row. How many chairs are in the classroom?

    A. 45

    B. 56

    C. 54

    D. 63

17) What number goes in the box to make the equation true?

$$\frac{\square}{5} = 2$$

    A. 8

    B. 10

    C. 16

    D. 32

18) Which number is represented by A?

    $13 \times A = 169$

    A. 9

    B. 10

    C. 13

    D. 12

19) What is the perimeter of this rectangle?

A. 12 cm

B. 24 cm

C. 32 cm

D. 64 cm

7 cm

5 cm ☐

20) Nicole has 3 quarters, 5 dimes, and 4 pennies. How much money does Nicole

have?

A. 155 pennies

B. 129 pennies

C. 255 pennies

D. 265 pennies

21) Noah packs 16 boxes with crayons. Each box holds 30 crayons. How many

crayons Noah can pack into these boxes?

A. 480

B. 540

C. 680

D. 720

22) A number sentence such as $88 - x = 28$ can be called an equation. If this equation is true, then which of the following equations is **NOT** true?

A. $88 - 28 = x$

B. $88 - x = 28$

C. $x - 28 = 88$

D. $x + 28 = 88$

23) There are 6 numbers in the box below. Which of the following list shows only even numbers from the numbers in the box?

13, 30, 46, 17, 82, 49

A. $13, 30, 46$

B. $13, 49, 82$

C. $13, 30, 82$

D. $30, 46, 82$

24) A cafeteria menu had spaghetti with meatballs for $10 and bean soup for $7. How much would it cost to buy five plates of spaghetti with meatballs and two bowls of bean soup?

A. 50

B. 64

C. 119

D. 350

25) Use the picture below to answer the question.

Which fraction shows the shaded part of this square?

A. $\frac{84}{100}$

B. $\frac{84}{10}$

C. $\frac{8.4}{100}$

D. $\frac{4}{100}$

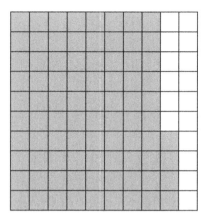

26) Use the table below to answer the question.

Based on their populations, which list of cities is in order from least to greatest?

A. Longview; Edinburg; Mission; Bryan

B. Bryan; Longview; Edinburg; Mission

C. Mission; Edinburg; Longview; Bryan

D. Bryan; Longview; Mission; Edinburg

City Populations	
City	Population
Bryan	78,087
Mission	78,807
Longview	78,108
Edinburg	78,708

27) Which number correctly completes the number sentence $20 \times 45 =$?

A. 225

B. 900

C. 1,250

D. 2,250

28) There are 60 minutes in an hour. How many minutes are in 5 hours?

    A. 300 minutes

    B. 320 minutes

    C. 360 minutes

    D. 400 minutes

29) Which number correctly completes the number sentence $52 \times 14 =$?

    A. 550

    B. 660

    C. 728

    D. 990

30) Michael has 845 marbles. What is this number rounded to the nearest ten?

    A. 850

    B. 840

    C. 800

    D. 8450

"This is the end of practice test 2"

Smarter Balanced Assessment Consortium (SBAC)

SBAC Practice Test 3

Mathematics

GRADE 3

- ❖ **30 Questions**
- ❖ **There is no time limit for this practice test.**
- ❖ **Calculators are NOT permitted for this practice test**

Administered *Month Year*

1) Classroom A contains 8 rows of chairs with 6 chairs per row. If classroom B has two times as many chairs, which number sentence can be used to find the number of chairs in classroom B?

A. $8 \times 6 + 2$

B. $8 + 6 \times 2$

C. $8 \times 6 \times 2$

D. $8 + 6 + 2$

2) There are 7 days in a week. There are 24 hours in day. How many hours are in a week?

A. 168

B. 196

C. 68

D. 28

3) Ella described a number using these clues:

Three-digit odd numbers that have a 9 in the hundreds place and a 5 in the tens place. Which number could fit Ella's description?

A. 949

B. 959

C. 958

D. 956

4) A cafeteria menu had spaghetti with meatballs for $9 and bean soup for $6

How much would it cost to buy three plates of spaghetti with meatballs and

three bowls of bean soup?

Write your answer in the box below.

5) This clock shows a time after 2:15 PM. What time was it 2 hours and 30

minutes ago?

A. 12:45 PM

B. 11:00 PM

C. 11:15 PM

D. 11:45 AM

6) A football team is buying new uniforms. Each uniform cost $50. The team

wants to buy 14 uniforms.

Which equation represents a way to find the total cost of the uniforms?

A. $(50 \times 10) + (1 \times 14) = 500 + 14$

B. $(50 \times 10) + (10 \times 1) = 500 + 10$

C. $(50 \times 10) + (50 \times 4) = 500 + 200$

D. $(14 \times 10) + (10 \times 20) = 140 + 200$

7) Olivia has 132 pastilles. She wants to put them in boxes of 4 pastilles. How many boxes does she need?

    A. 32

    B. 33

    C. 38

    D. 29

8) There are 76 students from Riddle Elementary school at the library on Tuesday. The other 48 students in the school are practicing in the classroom. Which number sentence shows the total number of students in Riddle Elementary school?

    A. $76 + 48$

    B. $76 - 48$

    C. 76×48

    D. $76 \div 48$

9) Martin earns There are 6 numbers in the box below. Which of the following list shows only odd numbers from the numbers in the box?

15, 40, 22, 16, 71, 33

    A. 15, 22, 16

    B. 15, 33, 71

    C. 15, 40, 22

    D. 22, 16, 40

10) Mia's goal is to save $157 to purchase her favorite bike.

- In January, she saved $52.

- In February, she saved $29.

How much money does Mia need to save in March to be able to purchase her favorite bike?

A. $29

B. $38

C. $55

D. $76

11) Michelle has 75 old books. She plans to send all of them to the library in their area. If she puts the books in boxes which can hold 5 books, which of the following equations can be used to find the number of boxes she will use?

A. $75 + 5 = $ _____

B. $75 \times 5 = $ _____

C. $75 - 5 = $ _____

D. $75 \div 5 = $ _____

12) Which number is made up of 8 hundred, 4 tens, and 9 ones?

A. 8,094

B. 849

C. 897

D. 498

13) Elise had 984 cards. Then, she gave 372 of the cards to her friend Alice.

After that, Elise lost 265 cards.

Which equation can be used to find the number of cards Elise has now?

A. $984 - 372 + 265 = $ _____

B. $984 - 372 - 265 = $ _____

C. $984 + 372 + 265 = $ _____

D. $984 + 372 - 265 = $ _____

14) The length of the following rectangle is 8 centimeters and its width is 6

centimeters. What is the area of the rectangle?

A. 14 cm^2

B. 28 cm^2

C. 48 cm^2

D. 32 cm^2

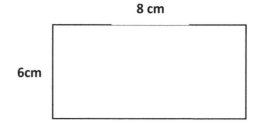

15) Look at the spinner above. On which color is the spinner most likely to

land?

A. Yellow

B. Green

C. Red

D. None

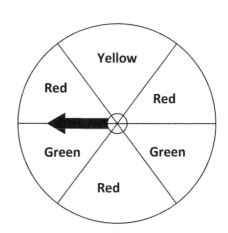

16) A group of third grade students recorded the following distances that they jumped.

25 inches	38 inches	26 inches	30 inches
38 inches	35 inches	27 inches	36 inches
34 inches	30 inches	36 inches	38 inches

What is the distance that was jumped most often?

A. 25

B. 26

C. 34

D. 38

17) Emma flew 5,288 miles from Los Angeles to New York City. What is the number of miles Emma flew rounded to the nearest thousand?

A. 4,000

B. 4,300

C. 4,500

D. 5,000

18) To what number is the arrow pointing?

A. 16

B. 14

C. 15

D. 12

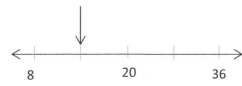

19) A number sentence such as 38 + Z = 84 can be called an equation. If this equation is true, then which of the following equations is not true?

A. 84 – 38 = Z

B. 84 – Z = 38

C. Z – 84 = 38

D. Z = 46

20) Use the picture below to answer the question. Which fraction shows the shaded part of this square?

A. $\frac{81}{100}$

B. $\frac{81}{10}$

C. $\frac{81}{1,000}$

D. $\frac{8}{100}$

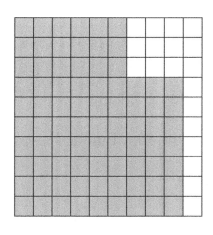

21) Which number correctly completes the number sentence 90 × 32 =?

A. 300

B. 800

C. 1,240

D. 2,880

22) Which number correctly completes the subtraction sentence

6,000 – 688 = _____?

A. 5,312

B. 3,482

C. 787

D. 5,152

23) Jason packs 14 boxes with flashcards. Each box holds 25 flashcards. How many flashcards Jason can pack into these boxes?

A. 76

B. 820

C. 520

D. 350

24) Which of the following statements describes the number 22,395?

A. The sum of two thousand, 2 thousand, five hundred, ninety tens, and five ones

B. The sum of twenty thousand, 2 thousand, five hundred, nine tens, and five ones

C. The sum of twenty thousand, 2 thousand, fifty hundred, ninety tens, and five ones

D. The sum of twenty thousand, 2 thousand, three hundred, nine tens, and five ones

25) The following models are the same size and each divided into equal parts.

The models can be used to write two fractions.

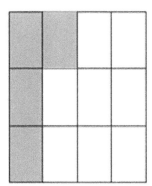 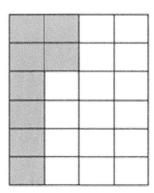

Based on the models, which of the following statements is true?

A. $\frac{4}{12}$ is bigger than $\frac{8}{24}$.

B. $\frac{4}{12}$ is smaller than $\frac{8}{24}$.

C. $\frac{4}{12}$ is equal to $\frac{8}{24}$.

D. We cannot compare these two fractions only by using the models.

26) What is the value of "A" in the following equation?

$$33 + A + 7 = 57$$

A. 15

B. 17

C. 13

D. 21

27) Emily has 126 stickers and she wants to give them to seven of her closest friends. If she gives them all an equal number of stickers, how many stickers will each of Emily's friends receive?

Write your answer in the box below.

28) Use the models below to answer the question.

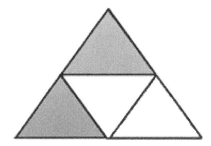 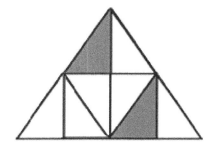

Which statement about the models is true?

A. Each shows the same fraction because they are the same size.

B. Each shows a different fraction because they are different shapes.

C. Each shows the same fraction because they both have 2 sections shaded.

D. Each shows a different fraction because they both have 2 shaded sections but a different number of total sections.

29) Mr. smith usually eats Three meals a day. How many meals does he eat in

a week?

A. 16

B. 21

C. 28

D. 33

30) What is the value of A in the equation $72 \div A = 9$?

A. 3

B. 5

C. 8

D. 7

"This is the end of the practice test 3"

Smarter Balanced Assessment Consortium (SBAC)

SBAC Practice Test 4

Mathematics

GRADE 3

- ❖ **30 Questions**
- ❖ **There is no time limit for this practice test.**
- ❖ **Calculators are NOT permitted for this practice test**

Administered *Month Year*

1) What number makes this equation true?

$$12 \times 8 = \square$$

  A. 86

  B. 96

  C. 106

  D. 68

2) Kayla has 140 red cards and 92 white cards. How many more reds cards than white cards do Kayla have?

  A. 27

  B. 18

  C. 48

  D. 28

3) A number sentence is shown below.

$$4 \times 6 \,\square\, 7 = 168$$

What symbol goes into the box to make the number sentence true?

  A. $\times$

  B. $\div$

  C. $+$

  D. $-$

4) Liam had 792 marbles. Then, he gave 328 of the cards to his friend Ethan.

After that, Liam lost 105 cards.

Which equation can be used to find the number of cards Eve has now?

A. 792 – 328 + 105 = ____

B. 792 – 328 – 105 = ____

C. 792 + 328 + 105 = ____

D. 792 + 328 – 105 = ____

5) What is the value of "B" in the following equation? $27 + B + 12 = 83$

A. 36

B. 28

C. 27

D. 44

6) There are two different cards on the table.

- There are 4 rows that have 8 red cards in each row.

- There are 19 white cards.

How many cards are there on the table?

A. 24

B. 51

C. 32

D. 92

7) Mason is 15 months now and he usually eats five meals a day. How many

meals does he eat in a week?

    A. 32

    B. 38

    C. 35

    D. 42

8) Which of the following list shows only fractions that are equivalent to $\frac{1}{4}$?

    A. $\frac{2}{8}, \frac{5}{20}, \frac{12}{48}$

    B. $\frac{6}{18}, \frac{5}{15}, \frac{4}{16}$

    C. $\frac{2}{8}, \frac{4}{16}, \frac{6}{18}$

    D. $\frac{2}{8}, \frac{5}{10}, \frac{12}{48}$

9) What mixed number is shown by the shaded triangles?

    A. $2\frac{1}{2}$

    B. $2\frac{1}{4}$

    C. $3\frac{1}{4}$

    D. $2\frac{3}{4}$

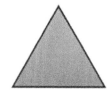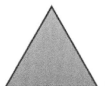

10) The perimeter of a square is 36 units. Each side of this square is the same

length. What is the length of one side of the square in units?

A. 4

B. 6

C. 8

D. 9

11) Which of the following comparison of fractions is true?

A. $\frac{2}{7} = \frac{4}{14}$

B. $\frac{2}{3} > \frac{4}{6}$

C. $\frac{2}{3} < \frac{4}{6}$

D. $\frac{4}{5} < \frac{2}{10}$

12) The sum of 6 ten thousand, 5 hundred, and 9 tens can be expressed as what

number in standard form?

A. 6,590

B. 60,590

C. 60,059

D. 60,509

13) One side of a square is 8 feet. What is the area of the square?

Write your answer in the box below.

14) What is the perimeter of the following triangle?

A. 45 inches

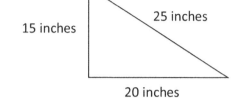

B. 30 inches

C. 60 inches

D. 150 inches

15) Moe has 750 cards. He wants to put them in boxes of 30 cards. How many

boxes does he need?

A. 24

B. 32

C. 28

D. 25

16) There are 9 rows of chairs in a classroom with 6 chairs in each row. How

many chairs are in the classroom?

A. 46

B. 54

C. 45

D. 64

17) What number goes in the box to make the equation true?

$$\frac{\Box}{6} = 3$$

A. 9

B. 18

C. 15

D. 63

18) Which number is represented by A?

$14 \times A = 196$

A. 12

B. 8

C. 14

D. 15

19) What is the perimeter of this rectangle?

A. 14 cm

B. 28 cm

C. 30 cm

D. 48 cm

8 cm

6 cm

20) Nicole has 4 quarters, 2 dimes, and 8 pennies. How much money does Nicole have?

A. 255 pennies

B. 128 pennies

C. 256 pennies

D. 182 pennies

21) Noah packs 18 boxes with crayons. Each box holds 25 crayons. How many crayons Noah can pack into these boxes?

A. 680

B. 540

C. 620

D. 450

22) A number sentence such as $74 - x = 54$ can be called an equation. If this equation is true, then which of the following equations is **NOT** true?

A. $74 - 54 = x$

B. $74 - x = 54$

C. $x - 54 = 74$

D. $x + 54 = 74$

23) There are 6 numbers in the box below. Which of the following list shows only even numbers from the numbers in the box?

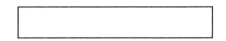

23, 32, 58, 27, 80, 41

A. 23, 32, 58

B. 23, 41, 80

C. 23, 32, 80

D. 58, 32, 80

24) A cafeteria menu had spaghetti with meatballs for $20 and bean soup for $6. How much would it cost to buy four plates of spaghetti with meatballs and three bowls of bean soup?

Write your answer in the box below.

25) Which number correctly completes the number sentence $15 \times 64 =$?

A. 220

B. 960

C. 1,200

D. 2,100

26) There are 60 minutes in an hour. How many minutes are in 3 hours?

   A. 180 minutes

   B. 300 minutes

   C. 108 minutes

   D. 200 minutes

27) Which number correctly completes the number sentence $47 \times 16 =$?

   A. 567

   B. 676

   C. 752

   D. 652

28) Michael has 675 marbles. What is this number rounded to the nearest ten?

   Write your answer in the box below.

29) Use the picture below to answer the question.

   Which fraction shows the shaded part of this square?

   A. $\frac{74}{100}$

   B. $\frac{74}{10}$

   C. $\frac{7.4}{100}$

   D. $\frac{7}{100}$

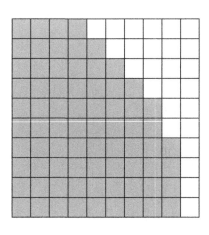

30) Use the table below to answer the question.

Based on their populations, which list of cities is in order from least to greatest?

A. Bryan; Edinburg; Longview; Mission

B. Bryan; Longview; Edinburg; Mission

C. Edinburg; Mission; Longview; Bryan

D. Longview; Edinburg; Mission; Bryan

City Populations	
City	Population
Bryan	65,056
Mission	65,605
Longview	65,305
Edinburg	65,506

"This is the end of practice test 4"

Smarter Balanced Assessment Consortium (SBAC)

SBAC Practice Test 5

Mathematics

GRADE 3

❖ **30 Questions**

❖ **There is no time limit for this practice test.**

❖ **Calculators are NOT permitted for this practice test**

Administered *Month Year*

1) Classroom A contains 5 rows of chairs with 4 chairs per row. If classroom B has three times as many chairs, which number sentence can be used to find the number of chairs in classroom B?

A. $5 \times 4 + 3$

B. $5 + 4 \times 3$

C. $5 \times 4 \times 3$

D. $5 + 4 + 3$

2) There are 7 days in a week. There are 24 hours in day. How many hours are in two weeks?

A. 336

B. 168

C. 320

D. 30

3) Ella described a number using these clues:

Three-digit odd numbers that have a 7 in the hundreds place and a 3 in the tens place. Which number could fit Ella's description?

A. 723

B. 735

C. 736

D. 734

4) A cafeteria menu had spaghetti with meatballs for $7 and bean soup for $5

How much would it cost to buy two plates of spaghetti with meatballs and

two bowls of bean soup?

Write your answer in the box below.

5) This clock shows a time after 8:15 PM. What time was it 3 hours and 35

minutes ago?

A. 05:40 PM

B. 05:05 PM

C. 04:45 PM

D. 04:40 PM

6) A football team is buying new uniforms. Each uniform cost $30. The team

wants to buy 12 uniforms.

Which equation represents a way to find the total cost of the uniforms?

A. $(30 \times 10) + (1 \times 12) = 300 + 12$

B. $(30 \times 10) + (12 \times 1) = 300 + 12$

C. $(30 \times 10) + (30 \times 2) = 300 + 60$

D. $(12 \times 10) + (10 \times 30) = 120 + 300$

7) Olivia has 120 pastilles. She wants to put them in boxes of 6 pastilles. How many boxes does she need?

A. 30

B. 20

C. 22

D. 19

8) There are 82 students from Riddle Elementary school at the library on Tuesday. The other 33 students in the school are practicing in the classroom. Which number sentence shows the total number of students in Riddle Elementary school?

A. $82 + 33$

B. $82 - 33$

C. 82×33

D. $82 \div 33$

9) Martin earns There are 6 numbers in the box below. Which of the following list shows only odd numbers from the numbers in the box?

19, 30, 18, 28, 83, 65

A. 19, 28, 18

B. 19, 65, 83

C. 19, 28, 28

D. 30, 18, 28

10) Mia's goal is to save $120 to purchase her favorite bike.

  - In January, she saved $40.

  - In February, she saved $25.

  How much money does Mia need to save in March to be able to purchase

  her favorite bike?

  A. $40

  B. $25

  C. $45

  D. $55

11) Michelle has 52 old books. She plans to send all of them to the library in

  their area. If she puts the books in boxes which can hold 4 books, which of

  the following equations can be used to find the number of boxes she will

  use?

  A. $52 + 4 = $ _____
  B. $52 \times 4 = $ _____
  C. $52 - 4 = $ _____
  D. $52 \div 4 = $ _____

12) Which number is made up of 6 hundred, 3 tens, and 5 ones?

  A. 6,053

  B. 635

  C. 653

  D. 356

13) Elise had 520 cards. Then, she gave 210 of the cards to her friend Alice.

 After that, Elise lost 110 cards.

 Which equation can be used to find the number of cards Elise has now?

 A. $520 - 210 + 110 =$ _____

 B. $520 - 210 - 110 =$ _____

 C. $520 + 210 + 110 =$ _____

 D. $520 + 210 - 110 =$ _____

14) The length of the following rectangle is 9 centimeters and its width is 5

 centimeters. What is the area of the rectangle?

 A. 15 cm^2

 B. 35cm^2

 C. 45 cm^2

 D. 28 cm^2

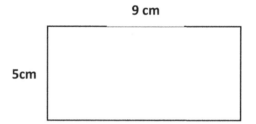

15) Look at the spinner above. On which color is the spinner most likely to

 land?

 A. Red

 B. Yellow

 C. Green

 D. None

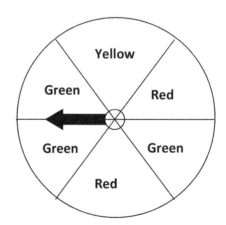

16) A group of third grade students recorded the following distances that they jumped.

22 inches	35 inches	23 inches	27 inches
35 inches	32 inches	24 inches	33 inches
31 inches	27 inches	33 inches	35 inches

What is the distance that was jumped most often?

A. 22

B. 23

C. 31

D. 35

17) Emma flew 3,124 miles from Los Angeles to New York City. What is the number of miles Emma flew rounded to the nearest thousand?

A. 4,100

B. 4,000

C. 3,100

D. 3,000

18) To what number is the arrow pointing?

A. 8

B. 7

C. 5

D. 6

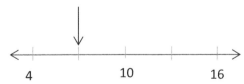

19) A number sentence such as 19 + Z = 42 can be called an equation. If this equation is true, then which of the following equations is not true?

    A. $42 - 19 = Z$

    B. $42 - Z = 19$

    C. $Z - 42 = 19$

    D. $Z = 23$

20) Use the picture below to answer the question. Which fraction shows the shaded part of this square?

    A. $\dfrac{74}{100}$

    B. $\dfrac{74}{10}$

    C. $\dfrac{74}{1,000}$

    D. $\dfrac{7}{100}$

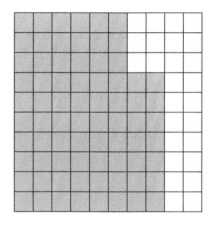

21) Which number correctly completes the number sentence $44 \times 25 =$?

    A. 810

    B. 950

    C. 1,050

    D. 1,100

22) Which number correctly completes the subtraction sentence

$3,000 - 237 =$ _____ ?

A. 2,763

B. 3,521

C. 835

D. 2,251

23) Jason packs 12 boxes with flashcards. Each box holds 18 flashcards. How many flashcards Jason can pack into these boxes?

A. 261

B. 621

C. 210

D. 216

24) Which of the following statements describes the number 34,678?

A. The sum of three thousand, 4 thousand, six hundred, seventy tens, and eight ones

B. The sum of forty thousand, 3 thousand, seven hundred, six tens, and eight ones

C. The sum of thirty thousand, 4 thousand, sixty hundred, seventy tens, and eight ones

D. The sum of thirty thousand, 4 thousand, six hundred, seven tens, and eight ones

25) The following models are the same size and each divided into equal parts.

The models can be used to write two fractions.

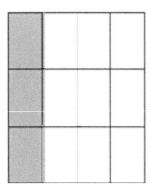 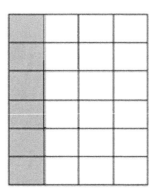

Based on the models, which of the following statements is true?

A. $\frac{3}{12}$ is bigger than $\frac{6}{24}$.

B. $\frac{3}{12}$ is smaller than $\frac{6}{24}$.

C. $\frac{3}{12}$ is equal to $\frac{6}{24}$.

D. We cannot compare these two fractions only by using the models.

26) What is the value of "A" in the following equation?

$$28 + A + 6 = 46$$

A. 13

B. 12

C. 14

D. 18

27) Emily has 90 stickers and she wants to give them to six of her closest

friends. If she gives them all an equal number of stickers, how many

stickers will each of Emily's friends receive?

Write your answer in the box below.

28) Use the models below to answer the question.

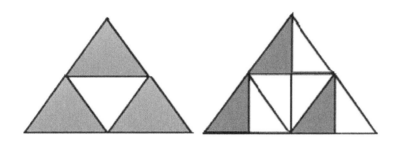

Which statement about the models is true?

A. Each shows the same fraction because they are the same size.

B. Each shows a different fraction because they are different shapes.

C. Each shows the same fraction because they both have 3 sections

shaded.

D. Each shows a different fraction because they both have 3 shaded

sections but a different number of total sections.

29) Mr. smith usually eats Two meals a day. How many meals does he eat in

a week?

A. 15

B. 14

C. 12

D. 21

30) What is the value of A in the equation $42 \div A = 7$?

A. 5

B. 7

C. 6

D. 9

"This is the end of the practice test 5"

Smarter Balanced Assessment Consortium (SBAC)

SBAC Practice Test 6

Mathematics

GRADE 3

❖ **30 Questions**

❖ **There is no time limit for this practice test.**

❖ **Calculators are NOT permitted for this practice test**

Administered *Month Year*

1) What number makes this equation true?

$$14 \times 6 = \square$$

   A. 82

   B. 84

   C. 98

   D. 56

2) Kayla has 110 red cards and 63 white cards. How many more reds cards than white cards do Kayla have?

   A. 137

   B. 173

   C. 47

   D. 74

3) A number sentence is shown below.

$$3 \times 5 \;\square\; 10 = 150$$

What symbol goes into the box to make the number sentence true?

   A. $\times$

   B. $\div$

   C. $+$

   D. $-$

4) Liam had 630 marbles. Then, he gave 250 of the cards to his friend Ethan.

 After that, Liam lost 85 cards.

 Which equation can be used to find the number of cards Eve has now?

 A. $630 - 250 + 85 =$

 B. $630 - 250 - 85 =$

 C. $630 + 250 + 85 =$

 D. $630 + 250 - 85 =$

5) What is the value of "B" in the following equation? $40 + B + 15 = 73$

 A. 32

 B. 56

 C. 16

 D. 18

6) There are two different cards on the table.

 - There are 3 rows that have 17 red cards in each row.

 - There are 14 white cards.

 How many cards are there on the table?

 A. 62

 B. 65

 C. 55

 D. 52

7) Mason is 15 months now and he usually eats two meals a day. How many

meals does he eat in a week?

    A. 12

    B. 18

    C. 14

    D. 16

8) Which of the following list shows only fractions that are equivalent to $\frac{1}{2}$?

    A. $\frac{2}{4}, \frac{7}{14}, \frac{5}{10}$

    B. $\frac{1}{3}, \frac{7}{14}, \frac{5}{10}$

    C. $\frac{5}{10}, \frac{7}{14}, \frac{4}{6}$

    D. $\frac{7}{14}, \frac{5}{10}, \frac{1}{4}$

9) What mixed number is shown by the shaded triangles?

    A. $2\frac{1}{4}$

    B. $2\frac{1}{2}$

    C. $3\frac{1}{2}$

    D. $1\frac{3}{4}$

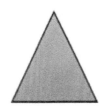

10) The perimeter of a square is 24 units. Each side of this square is the same

length. What is the length of one side of the square in units?

A. 3

B. 8

C. 6

D. 5

11) Which of the following comparison of fractions is true?

A. $\frac{1}{5} = \frac{1}{6}$

B. $\frac{1}{4} > \frac{3}{4}$

C. $\frac{3}{7} < \frac{5}{7}$

D. $\frac{3}{9} < \frac{1}{9}$

12) The sum of 4 ten thousand, 3 hundred, and 7 tens can be expressed as what

number in standard form?

A. 4,370

B. 40,370

C. 40,037

D. 40,307

13) One side of a square is 6 feet. What is the area of the square?

Write your answer in the box below.

14) What is the perimeter of the following triangle?

A. 30 inches

B. 28 inches

C. 36 inches

D. 54 inches

9 inches   15 inches

12 inches

15) Moe has 500 cards. He wants to put them in boxes of 25 cards. How many boxes does he need?

A. 22

B. 18

C. 26

D. 20

16) There are 7 rows of chairs in a classroom with 5 chairs in each row. How many chairs are in the classroom?

A. 30

B. 35

C. 32

D. 24

17) What number goes in the box to make the equation true?

$$\frac{\square}{3} = 4$$

   A. 8

   B. 12

   C. 14

   D. 16

18) Which number is represented by A?

$12 \times A = 144$

   A. 15

   B. 9

   C. 12

   D. 13

19) What is the perimeter of this rectangle?

   A. 13 cm

   B. 22 cm

   C. 28 cm

   D. 24 cm

7 cm

4 cm

20) Nicole has 2 quarters, 3 dimes, and 5 pennies. How much money does Nicole have?

A. 80 pennies

B. 85 pennies

C. 70 pennies

D. 75 pennies

21) Noah packs 30 boxes with crayons. Each box holds 14 crayons. How many crayons Noah can pack into these boxes?

A. 480

B. 520

C. 510

D. 420

22) A number sentence such as $67 - x = 36$ can be called an equation. If this equation is true, then which of the following equations is **NOT** true?

A. $63 - 36 = X$

B. $67 - X = 36$

C. $X - 36 = 67$

D. $X + 36 = 67$

23) There are 6 numbers in the box below. Which of the following list shows only even numbers from the numbers in the box?

13, 22, 48, 17, 70, 31

A. 13, 22, 48

B. 13, 31, 70

C. 13, 22, 70

D. 48, 22, 70

24) A cafeteria menu had spaghetti with meatballs for $15 and bean soup for $5. How much would it cost to buy five plates of spaghetti with meatballs and two bowls of bean soup?

Write your answer in the box below.

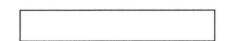

25) Which number correctly completes the number sentence $12 \times 55 =$?

A. 620

B. 660

C. 1,320

D. 1,200

26) There are 60 minutes in an hour. How many minutes are in 2 hours?

   A. 120 minutes

   B. 200 minutes

   C. 360 minutes

   D. 140 minutes

27) Which number correctly completes the number sentence $32 \times 15 =$?

   A. 520

   B. 580

   C. 480

   D. 420

28) Michael has 547 marbles. What is this number rounded to the nearest ten?

   Write your answer in the box below.

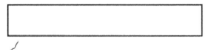

29) Use the picture below to answer the question.

   Which fraction shows the shaded part of this square?

   A. $\dfrac{72}{100}$

   B. $\dfrac{72}{10}$

   C. $\dfrac{7.2}{100}$

   D. $\dfrac{0.72}{100}$

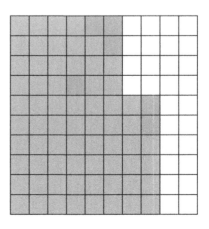

30) Use the table below to answer the question.

Based on their populations, which list of cities is in order from least to greatest?

A. Bryan; Edinburg; Longview; Mission

B. Bryan; Longview; Edinburg; Mission

C. Edinburg; Mission; Longview; Bryan

D. Longview; Edinburg; Mission; Bryan

City Populations	
City	Population
Bryan	14,021
Mission	14,905
Longview	14,206
Edinburg	14,408

"This is the end of practice test 6"

Answers and Explanations

SBAC Practice Tests

❋ Now, it's time to review your results to see where you went wrong and what areas you need to improve!

SBAC - Mathematics

Practice Test - 1						Practice Test - 2					
1	B	11	D	21	D	1	C	11	A	21	A
2	A	12	B	22	A	2	A	12	B	22	C
3	B	13	B	23	D	3	B	13	C	23	D
4	C	14	C	24	D	4	B	14	C	24	B
5	A	15	C	25	C	5	C	15	D	25	A
6	B	16	D	26	B	6	A	16	B	26	B
7	C	17	D	27	A	7	B	17	B	27	B
8	D	18	B	28	D	8	D	18	C	28	A
9	C	19	C	29	B	9	B	19	B	29	C
10	D	20	A	30	C	10	D	20	B	30	A

SBAC - Mathematics

Practice Test - 3					
1	C	11	D	21	D
2	A	12	B	22	A
3	B	13	B	23	D
4	45	14	C	24	D
5	D	15	C	25	C
6	C	16	D	26	B
7	B	17	D	27	18
8	A	18	B	28	D
9	B	19	C	29	B
10	D	20	A	30	C

Practice Test - 4					
1	B	11	A	21	D
2	C	12	B	22	C
3	A	13	64	23	D
4	B	14	C	24	98
5	D	15	D	25	B
6	B	16	B	26	A
7	C	17	B	27	C
8	A	18	C	28	680
9	B	19	B	29	A
10	D	20	B	30	B

SBAC - Mathematics

Practice Test - 5

#		#		#	
1	C	11	D	21	D
2	A	12	B	22	A
3	B	13	B	23	D
4	24	14	C	24	D
5	D	15	C	25	C
6	C	16	D	26	B
7	B	17	D	27	15
8	A	18	B	28	D
9	B	19	C	29	B
10	D	20	A	30	C

Practice Test - 6

#		#		#	
1	B	11	C	21	D
2	C	12	B	22	C
3	A	13	36	23	D
4	B	14	C	24	85
5	D	15	D	25	B
6	B	16	B	26	A
7	C	17	B	27	C
8	A	18	C	28	550
9	B	19	B	29	A
10	D	20	B	30	B

Answers and

Explanations

Practice Test 1

SBAC - Mathematics

Answers and Explanations

1) Answer: B.

Olivia wants to put 93 pastilles into boxes of 3 pastilles. Therefore, she needs ($93 \div 3 =$) 31 boxes.

2) Answer: A.

To find the total number of students in Riddle Elementary School, add 82 with 64.

3) Answer: B.

An easy way to tell whether a large number is odd or even is to look at its final digit. If the number ends with an odd digit (1, 3, 5, 7, or 9), then it's odd. On the other hand, if the number ends with an even digit or 0 (0, 2, 4, 6 or 8), then it is even.

13, 39 and 73 ends with odd digit, therefore, they are odd numbers.

4) Answer: C.

Classroom A contains 7 rows of chairs with four chairs per row. Therefore, there are ($7 \times 5 =$) 35 chairs in Classroom A. Classroom B has three times as many chairs. Then, there are ($7 \times 5 \times 3$) chairs in Classroom B.

5) Answer: A.

1 day: 24 hours

2 days = $2 \times 24 = 48$ hours

6) Answer: B.

Three-digit odd numbers that have a 7 in the hundreds place and a 3 in the tens place is 737. 732 and 736 are even numbers.

7) Answer: C.

3 plates of spaghetti with meatballs cost: $3 \times \$8 = \$24$

3 bowls of bean soup cost: $3 \times \$7 = \$21$

3 plates of spaghetti with meatballs + 3 bowls of bean soup cost:

$\$24 + \$21 = \$45$

8) Answer: D.

The clock shows 2:15 PM. One hour before that was 1:15 PM. 45 minutes before that was 12:30 PM.

9) Answer: C.

The Football team buys 12 uniforms that each uniform cost $30. Therefore, they should pay $(12 \times \$30 =)$ $360.

Choice C is the correct answer. $(30 \times 10) + (30 \times 2) = 300 + 60 = 360$

10) Answer: D.

Mia saved $46 and $38. Therefore, she has $84 now.

$\$160 - \$84 = \$76$. She needs to save 76.

11) Answer: D.

Michelle puts 84 books in 4 boxes. Therefore, $84 \div 4$ formula is correct.

12) Answer: B.

To find the number, put 5 for hundreds place, 7 for tens place, and 6 for ones place. Then, you will get: $500 + 70 + 6 = 576$

13) Answer: B.

Elise gave 352 of her 956 cards to her friend. Therefore, she has $956 - 352$ cards now. Then she lost 250 cards. Now, she has $(956 - 352 - 250) = 354$ cards

14) Answer: C.

Use area formula of a rectangle: Area = length × width

Area = 4cm × 9cm = 36 cm^2

15) Answer: C.

The chance of landing on yellow is 3 out of 6.

The chance of landing on red is 1 out of 6.

The chance of landing on green is 2 out of 6.

The chance of landing on yellow red is more than the chance of landing on other colors.

16) Answer: D.

36 is the most frequent number in the table.

17) Answer: D.

The number 3,391 rounded to the nearest thousand is 3,000.

18) Answer: B.

The arrow shows a number between two numbers 20 and 36. ($36 - 20 = 16, 16 \div 2 = 8$) $\Rightarrow 20 + 8 = 28$

Therefore, the answer is 28.

19) Answer: C.

$25 + Z = 92$. Then, $Z = (92 - 25 =) 67$.

All these equations are true:

$92 - 25 = Z$

$92 - Z = 25$

$Z = 67$

But this equation is not true: $Z - 92 = 25$

20) Answer: A.

The table is divided into 100 equal parts. 87 parts of these 100 parts are shaded. The shaded part is equal to $\frac{87}{100}$.

21) Answer: D.

$80 \times 35 = 2,800$

22) Answer: A.

$7,000 - 858 = 6,142$

23) Answer: D.

To find the answer, multiply 12 by 30. $12 \times 30 = 360$

24) Answer: D.

26,586 is the sum of: $20,000 + 6,000 + 500 + 80 + 6$

25) Answer: C.

The first model is divided into 12 equal parts. 3 out of 12 parts are shaded. That means $\frac{3}{12}$ which is equal to: $\frac{1}{4}$

The second model is divided into 24 equal parts. 6 out of 24 parts are shaded. That means $\frac{6}{24}$ which is equal to: $\frac{1}{4}$

26) Answer: B.

$A = 42 - 23 - 8 = 11$

27) Answer A.

$144 \div 9 = 16$

28) Answer: D.

The first model from left is divided into 4 equal parts. 3 out of 4 parts are shaded. The fraction for this model is $\frac{3}{4}$. The second model is divided into 8 equal parts. 3 out of 8 parts are shaded. Therefore, the fraction of the shaded parts for this model is $\frac{3}{8}$. These two models represent different fractions.

29) Answer: B.

2 meals a day, means $(2 \times 7 =)$ 14 meals a week.

30) Answer: C.

$A = 56 \div 8 = 7$

Practice Test 2

SBAC - Mathematics

Answers and Explanations

1) Answer: C.

If Mason eats 4 meals in 1 day, then, in a week (7 days) he eats ($7 \times 4 = 28$) meals.

2) Answer: A.

All these fractions; $\frac{3}{9}, \frac{5}{15}, \frac{24}{72}$ are equivalent to $\frac{1}{3}$.

3) Answer: B.

This shape shows 2 complete shaded rectangle and 3 parts of a triangle divided into 4 equal parts. It is equal to $2\frac{3}{4}$.

4) Answer: B.

$13 \times 5 = 65$

5) Answer: C.

To find the answer subtract 88 from 109. The answer is ($120 - 85$) = 35.

6) Answer: A.

$3 \times 5 = 15$. Then:

$3 \times 5 \square 8 = 120$

$15 \square 8 = 120 \Rightarrow 120 = 15 \times 8$

7) Answer: B.

Liam gave 432 of his marbles to his friend. Now he has $835 - 432 = 403$

He lost 116 of his marbles. Now, he has $403 - 116 = 287$ or ($835 - 432 - 116$).

8) Answer: D.

$43 + B + 7 = 63 \Rightarrow 50 + B = 63 \Rightarrow B = 63 - 50 = 13$

9) Answer: B.

3 rows that have 12 red cards in each row contain: $3 \times 12 = 36$ red cards

And there are 21 white cards on table. Therefore, there are $36 + 21 = 57$ cards on table.

10) Answer: D.

Perimeter of the square is 32. Then:

$32 = 4 \times \text{side} \Rightarrow \text{side} = 8$

Each side of the square is 8 units.

11) Answer: A.

Simplify $\frac{9}{15}$ that's equal to $\frac{3}{5}$. Only option A is correct.

12) Answer: B.

4 ten thousand = 40,000

7 hundred = 700

8 tens = 80

Add all: $40,000 + 700 + 80 = 40,780$

13) Answer: C.

To find the area of a square, multiply one side by itself.

Area of a square = (side) × (side) = $5 \times 5 = 25$

14) Answer: C.

To find the perimeter of the triangle, add all three sides.

Perimeter = $12 + 16 + 20 = 48$ inches

15) Answer: D.

Moe wants to put 460 cards into boxes of 20 cards. Therefore, he needs $(460 \div 20 =) 23$ boxes.

16) Answer: B.

8rows of chairs with 7 chairs in each row means: $8 \times 7 = 56$ chairs in total.

17) Answer: B.

We need to find a number that when divided by 5, the answer is 2.

Therefore, we are looking for 10.

18) Answer: C.

$A = 169 \div 13 \Rightarrow A = 13$

19) Answer: B.

Use perimeter of rectangle formula.

Perimeter $= 2 \times$ length $+ 2 \times$ width $\Rightarrow$ P$= 2 \times 5 + 2 \times 7 = 10 + 14 = 24$ cm

20) Answer: B.

3 quarters $= 3 \times 25$ pennies $= 75$ pennies

5 dimes $= 5 \times 10$ pennies $= 50$ pennies

In total Nicole has 129 pennies

21) Answer: A.

$16 \times 30 = 480$

22) Answer: C.

$88 - x = 28$. Then, $x = 88 - 28 = 60$

Let's review the equations provided:

A. $88 - 28 = x$ This is true!

B. $88 - x = 28$ This is true!

C. $x - 28 = 88$ This is NOT true!

D. $x + 28 = 88$ This is true!

23) Answer: D.

Even numbers always end with a digit 0, 2, 4, 6 or 8.

Therefore, numbers 30, 46, 82 are the only even numbers.

24) Answer: B.

5 spaghetti with meatballs cost: $5 \times \$10 = \$50$

2 bowls of bean soup cost: $2 \times \$7 = \$14$

5 spaghetti with meatballs + 2 bowls of bean soup cost: $50 + $ 14 = $64

25) Answer: A.

The table is divided into 100 equal parts. 88 parts of these 100 parts are shaded. It means $\frac{84}{100}$.

26) Answer: B.

Bryan city with 78,087 has the least population. Longview, Edinburg and Mission are other cities in order from least to greatest.

27) Answer: B.

$20 \times 45 = 900$

28) Answer: A.

1 hour = 60 minutes

5 hours = 5 × 60 minutes ⇒ 5hours = 300 minutes

29) Answer: C.

$52 \times 14 = 728$

30) Answer: A.

We round the number up to the nearest ten if the last digit in the number is 5, 6, 7, 8, or 9.

We round the number down to the nearest ten if the last digit in the number is 1, 2, 3, or 4.

If the last digit is 0, then we do not have to do any rounding, because it is already rounded to the ten.

Therefore, rounded number of 845 to the nearest ten is 850.

Practice Test 3

SBAC - Mathematics

Answers and Explanations

1) **Answer: C.**

Classroom A contains 8 rows of chairs with six chairs per row. Therefore, there are $(8 \times 6 =)$ 48 chairs in Classroom A. Classroom B has two times as many chairs. Then, there are $(8 \times 6 \times 2)$ chairs in Classroom B.

2) **Answer: A.**

1 day: 24 hours

7 days = $7 \times 24 = 168$ hours

3) **Answer: B.**

Three-digit odd numbers that have a 9 in the hundreds place and a 5 in the tens place is 959. 954 and 958 are even numbers.

4) **Answer: 45.**

3 plates of spaghetti with meatballs cost: $3 \times \$9 = \$27$

3 bowls of bean soup cost: $3 \times \$6 = \$18$

3 plates of spaghetti with meatballs + 3 bowls of bean soup cost: $\$27 + \$18 = \$45$

5) **Answer: D.**

The clock shows 2:15 PM. 2 hours before that was 12:15 AM. 30 minutes before that was 11:45 AM.

6) **Answer: C.**

The Football team buys 14 uniforms that each uniform cost $50. Therefore, they should pay $(14 \times \$50 =)$ $700.

Choice C is the correct answer. $(50 \times 10) + (50 \times 4) = 500 + 200 = 700$

7) **Answer: B.**

Olivia wants to put 132 pastilles into boxes of 4 pastilles.

Therefore, she needs $(132 \div 4 =)$ 33 boxes.

8) Answer: A.

To find the total number of students in Riddle Elementary School, add 76 with 48.

9) Answer: B.

An easy way to tell whether a large number is odd or even is to look at its final digit. If the number ends with an odd digit (1, 3, 5, 7, or 9), then it's odd. On the other hand, if the number ends with an even digit or 0 (0, 2, 4, 6 or 8), then it is even.

15, 33 and 71 ends with odd digit, therefore, they are odd numbers.

10) Answer: D.

Mia saved $52 and $29. Therefore, she has $81 now.

$157 - $81 = $76. She needs to save 76.

11) Answer: D.

Michelle puts 75 books in 5 boxes. Therefore, $75 \div 5$ formula is correct.

12) Answer: B.

To find the number, put 8 for hundreds place, 4 for tens place, and 9 for one's place. Then, you will get: $800 + 40 + 9 = 849$

13) Answer: B.

Elise gave 372 of her 984 cards to her friend. Therefore, she has $984 - 372$ cards now. Then she lost 265 cards. Now, she has $(984 - 372 - 265) = 347$ cards

14) Answer: C.

Use area formula of a rectangle:

Area = length × width

Area = 6cm × 8cm = 48 cm^2

15) Answer: C.

The chance of landing on red is 3 out of 6.

The chance of landing on yellow is 1 out of 6.

The chance of landing on green is 2 out of 6.

The chance of landing on red is more than the chance of landing on other colors.

16) Answer: D.

38 is the most frequent number in the table.

17) Answer: D.

The number 5,288 rounded to the nearest thousand is 5,000.

18) Answer: B.

The arrow shows a number between two numbers 8 and 20. ($20 - 8 = 12, 12 \div 2 = 6$) $\Longrightarrow 6 + 8 = 14$

Therefore, the answer is 14.

19) Answer: C.

$38 + Z = 84$. Then, $Z = (84 - 38=)$ 46.

All these equations are true:

$84 - 38 = Z$

$84 - Z = 38$

$Z = 46$

But this equation is not true: $Z - 84 = 38$

20) Answer: A.

The table is divided into 100 equal parts. 81 parts of these 100 parts are shaded.

The shaded part is equal to $\frac{81}{100}$.

21) Answer: D.

$90 \times 32 = 2,880$

22) Answer: A.

$6,000 - 688 = 5,312$

23) Answer: D.

To find the answer, multiply 14 by 25.

$14 \times 25 = 350$

24) Answer: D.

22,395 is the sum of:

$20,000 + 2,000 + 300 + 90 + 5$

25) Answer: C.

The first model is divided into 12 equal parts. 4 out of 12 parts are shaded. That means $\frac{4}{12}$ which is equal to: $\frac{1}{3}$

The second model is divided into 24 equal parts. 8 out of 24 parts are shaded. That means $\frac{8}{24}$ which is equal to: $\frac{1}{3}$

26) Answer: B.

$A = 57 - 33 - 7 = 17$

27) Answer 18.

$126 \div 7 = 18$

28) Answer: D.

The first model from left is divided into 4 equal parts. 2 out of 4 parts are shaded. The fraction for this model is $\frac{1}{2}$. The second model is divided into 8 equal parts. 2 out of 8 parts are shaded. Therefore, the fraction of the shaded parts for this model is $\frac{1}{4}$. These two models represent different fractions.

29) Answer: B.

3 meals a day, means $(3 \times 7 =) 21$ meals a week.

30) Answer: C.

$A = 72 \div 9 = 8$

Practice Test 4

SBAC - Mathematics

Answers and Explanations

1) Answer: B.

$12 \times 8 = 96$

2) Answer: C.

To find the answer subtract 92 from 140. The answer is $(140 - 92) = 48$.

3) Answer: A.

$4 \times 6 = 24$. Then: $4 \times 6 \; \square \; 7 = 168$

$24 \; \square \; 7 = 168 \Rightarrow 168 = 24 \times 7$

4) Answer: B.

Liam gave 328 of his marbles to his friend. Now he has $792 - 328 = 464$

He lost 105 of his marbles. Now, he has $464 - 105 = 359$ or $(729 - 328 - 105)$.

5) Answer: D.

$27 + B + 12 = 83 \Rightarrow 39 + B = 83 \Rightarrow B = 83 - 39 = 44$

6) Answer: B.

4 rows that have 8 red cards in each row contain: $4 \times 8 = 32$ red cards

And there are 19 white cards on table. Therefore, there are $32 + 19 = 51$ cards on table.

7) Answer: C.

If Mason eats 5 meals in 1 day, then, in a week (7days) he eats $(7 \times 5 = 35)$ meals.

8) Answer: A.

All these fractions; $\frac{2}{8}, \frac{5}{20}, \frac{12}{48}$ are equivalent to $\frac{1}{4}$.

9) Answer: B.

This shape shows 2 complete shaded triangles and 1 parts of a triangle divided into 4 equal parts. It is equal to $2\frac{1}{4}$.

10) Answer: D.

Perimeter of the square is 36. Then:

$36 = 4 \times \text{side} \Rightarrow \text{side} = 9$

Each side of the square is 9 units.

11) Answer: A.

Simplify $\frac{4}{14}$ that's equal to $\frac{2}{7}$. Only option A is correct.

12) Answer: B.

6 ten thousand = 60,000

5 hundred = 500

9 tens = 90

Add all: 60,000 + 500 + 90 = 60,590

13) Answer: 64.

To find the area of a square, multiply one side by itself.

Area of a square = (side) × (side) = 8 × 8 = 64

14) Answer: C.

To find the perimeter of the triangle, add all three sides.

Perimeter = 15 + 20 + 25 = 60 inches

15) Answer: D.

Moe wants to put 750 cards into boxes of 30 cards. Therefore, he needs (750 ÷ 30 =) 25 boxes.

16) Answer: B.

9 rows of chairs with 6 chairs in each row means: 9 × 6 = 54 chairs in total.

17) Answer: B.

We need to find a number that when divided by 6, the answer is 3. Therefore, we are looking for 18.

18) Answer: C.

$A = 196 \div 14 \Rightarrow A = 14$

19) Answer: B.

Use perimeter of rectangle formula.

Perimeter $= 2 \times$ length $+ 2 \times$ width $\Rightarrow$ P$= 2 \times 6 + 2 \times 8 = 12 + 16 = 28$ cm

20) Answer: B.

4 quarters $= 4 \times 25$ pennies $= 100$ pennies

2 dimes $= 2 \times 10$ pennies $= 20$ pennies

In total Nicole has 128 pennies

21) Answer: D.

$18 \times 25 = 450$

22) Answer: C.

$74 - x = 54$

Then, $x = 74 - 54 = 20$

Let's review the equations provided:

A. $74 - 54 = x$ This is true!

B. $74 - x = 54$ This is true!

C. $x - 54 = 74$ This is NOT true!

D. $x + 54 = 74$ This is true!

23) Answer: D.

Even numbers always end with a digit 0, 2, 4, 6 or 8.

Therefore, numbers 58, 32, 80 are the only even numbers.

24) Answer: 98.

4 spaghettis with meatballs cost: $4 \times \$20 = \$80$

3 bowls of bean soup cost: $3 \times \$6 = \$18$

4 spaghettis with meatballs + 3 bowls of bean soup cost: $\$80 + \$18 = \$98$

25) Answer: B.

$15 \times 64 = 960$

26) Answer: A.

1 hour $= 60$ minutes

3 hours $= 3 \times 60$ minutes $\Rightarrow$ 3hours $= 180$ minutes

27) Answer: C.

$47 \times 16 = 752$

28) Answer: 680.

We round the number up to the nearest ten if the last digit in the number is 5, 6, 7, 8, or 9.

We round the number down to the nearest ten if the last digit in the number is 1, 2, 3, or 4.

If the last digit is 0, then we do not have to do any rounding, because it is already rounded to the ten.

Therefore, rounded number of 675 to the nearest ten is 680.

29) Answer: A.

The table is divided into 100 equal parts. 74 parts of these 100 parts are shaded. It means $\frac{74}{100}$.

30) Answer: B.

Bryan city with 65,056 has the least population. Longview, Edinburg and Mission are other cities in order from least to greatest.

Practice Test 5

SBAC - Mathematics

Answers and Explanations

1) Answer: C.

Classroom A contains 5 rows of chairs with four chairs per row. Therefore, there are (5 × 4 =) 20 chairs in Classroom A. Classroom B has three times as many chairs. Then, there are (5 × 4 × 3) chairs in Classroom B.

2) Answer: A.

1 day: 24 hours

7 days = 7 × 24 = 168 hours, for two weeks: 2 × 168 = 336

3) Answer: B.

Three-digit odd numbers that have a 7 in the hundreds place and a 3 in the tens place is 735. 734 and 738 are even numbers.

4) Answer: 24.

2 plates of spaghetti with meatballs cost: 2 × $7 = $14

2 bowls of bean soup cost: 2 × $5 = $10

2 plates of spaghetti with meatballs + 2 bowls of bean soup cost: $14 + $10 = $24

5) Answer: D.

The clock shows 8:15 PM. 3 hours before that was 5:15 PM. 35 minutes before that was 4:40 PM.

6) Answer: C.

The Football team buys 12 uniforms that each uniform cost $30. Therefore, they should pay (12 × $30 =) $360.

Choice C is the correct answer. (30 × 10) + (30 × 2) = 300 + 60 = 360

7) Answer: B.

Olivia wants to put 120 pastilles into boxes of 6 pastilles.

Therefore, she needs (120 ÷ 6 =) 20 boxes.

8) Answer: A.

To find the total number of students in Riddle Elementary School, add 82 with 33.

9) Answer: B.

An easy way to tell whether a large number is odd or even is to look at its final digit. If the number ends with an odd digit (1, 3, 5, 7, or 9), then it's odd. On the other hand, if the number ends with an even digit or 0 (0, 2, 4, 6 or 8), then it is even.

19, 83 and 65 ends with odd digit, therefore, they are odd numbers.

10) Answer: D.

Mia saved $40 and $25. Therefore, she has $65 now.

$120 – $65 = $55. She needs to save 55.

11) Answer: D.

Michelle puts 52 books in 4 boxes. Therefore, $52 \div 4$ formula is correct.

12) Answer: B.

To find the number, put 6 for hundreds place, 3 for tens place, and 5 for one's place. Then, you will get: $600 + 30 + 5 = 635$

13) Answer: B.

Elise gave 210 of her 520 cards to her friend. Therefore, she has $520 – 210$ cards now. Then she lost 110 cards. Now, she has $(520 – 210 – 110) = 200$ cards

14) Answer: C.

Use area formula of a rectangle: Area = length × width

Area = 5cm × 9cm = 45 cm^2

15) Answer: C.

The chance of landing on red is 2 out of 6.

The chance of landing on yellow is 1 out of 6.

The chance of landing on green is 3 out of 6.

The chance of landing on green is more than the chance of landing on other colors.

16) Answer: D.

35 is the most frequent number in the table.

17) Answer: D.

The number 3,124 rounded to the nearest thousand is 3,000.

18) Answer: B.

The arrow shows a number between two numbers 4 and 10. $(10 - 4 = 6, 6 \div 2 = 3) \Longrightarrow 4 + 3 = 7$

Therefore, the answer is 7.

19) Answer: C.

$19 + Z = 42$. Then, $Z = (42 - 19 =)\ 23$.

All these equations are true:

$42 - 19 = Z$

$42 - Z = 19$

$Z = 23$

But this equation is not true: $Z - 42 = 19$

20) Answer: A.

The table is divided into 100 equal parts. 74 parts of these 100 parts are shaded.

The shaded part is equal to $\frac{74}{100}$.

21) Answer: D.

$44 \times 25 = 1,100$

22) Answer: A.

$3,000 - 237 = 2,763$

23) Answer: D.

To find the answer, multiply 12 by 18.

$12 \times 18 = 216$

24) Answer: D.

34,678 is the sum of:

$30,000 + 4,000 + 600 + 70 + 8$

25) Answer: C.

The first model is divided into 12 equal parts. 3 out of 12 parts are shaded. That means $\frac{3}{12}$ which is equal to: $\frac{1}{4}$

The second model is divided into 24 equal parts. 6 out of 24 parts are shaded. That means $\frac{6}{24}$ which is equal to: $\frac{1}{4}$

26) Answer: B.

$A = 46 - 28 - 6 = 12$

27) Answer 15.

$90 \div 6 = 15$

28) Answer: D.

The first model from left is divided into 4 equal parts. 3 out of 4 parts are shaded. The fraction for this model is $\frac{3}{4}$. The second model is divided into 8 equal parts. 3 out of 8 parts are shaded. Therefore, the fraction of the shaded parts for this model is $\frac{3}{8}$. These two models represent different fractions.

29) Answer: B.

2 meals a day, means $(2 \times 7 =)$ 14 meals a week.

30) Answer: C.

$A = 42 \div 7 = 6$

Practice Test 6

SBAC - Mathematics

Answers and Explanations

1) Answer: B.

$14 \times 6 = 84$

2) Answer: C.

To find the answer subtract 63 from 110. The answer is $(110 - 63) = 47$.

3) Answer: A.

$3 \times 5 = 15$. Then: $3 \times 5 \,\square\, 10 = 150$

$15 \,\square\, 10 = 150 \Rightarrow 150 = 15 \times 10$

4) Answer: B.

Liam gave 250 of his marbles to his friend. Now he has $630 - 250 = 380$

He lost 85 of his marbles. Now, he has $380 - 85 = 295$ or $(630 - 250 - 85)$.

5) Answer: D.

$40 + B + 15 = 73 \Rightarrow 55 + B = 73 \Rightarrow B = 73 - 55 = 18$

6) Answer: B.

3 rows that have 17 red cards in each row contain: $3 \times 17 = 51$ red cards

And there are 14 white cards on table. Therefore, there are $51 + 14 = 65$ cards on table.

7) Answer: C.

If Mason eats 2 meals in 1 day, then, in a week (7days) he eats $(7 \times 2 = 14)$ meals.

8) Answer: A.

All these fractions $\frac{2}{4}, \frac{7}{14}, \frac{5}{10}$ are equivalent to $\frac{1}{2}$.

9) Answer: B.

This shape shows 2 complete shaded triangles and 2 parts of a triangle divided into 4 equal parts. It is equal to $2\frac{1}{2}$.

10) Answer: D.

Perimeter of the square is 24. Then:

$24 = 4 \times$ side $\Rightarrow$ side $= 6$

Each side of the square is 6 units.

11) Answer: C.

Only option C is correct.

12) Answer: B.

4 ten thousand = 40,000

3 hundred = 300

7 tens = 70

Add all: 40,000 + 300 + 70 = 40,370

13) Answer: 36.

To find the area of a square, multiply one side by itself.

Area of a square = (side) $\times$ (side) = $6 \times 6 = 36$

14) Answer: C.

To find the perimeter of the triangle, add all three sides.

Perimeter = 9 + 12 + 15 = 36 inches

15) Answer: D.

Moe wants to put 500 cards into boxes of 25 cards. Therefore, he needs (500 ÷ 25 =) 20 boxes.

16) Answer: B.

7 rows of chairs with 5 chairs in each row means: $7 \times 5 = 35$ chairs in total.

17) Answer: B.

We need to find a number that when divided by 3, the answer is 4. Therefore, we are looking for 12.

18) Answer: C.

$A = 144 \div 12 \Rightarrow A = 12$

19) Answer: B.

Use perimeter of rectangle formula.

Perimeter = 2 × length + 2 × width ⟹ P= 2 × 4 + 2 × 7 = 8 +14 = 22 cm

20) Answer: B.

2 quarters = 2 × 25 pennies = 50 pennies

3 dimes = 3 × 10 pennies = 30 pennies

In total Nicole has 85 pennies

21) Answer: D.

$30 \times 14 = 420$

22) Answer: C.

$67 - x = 36$

Then, $x = 67 - 36 = 31$

Let's review the equations provided:

A. $67 - 36 = x$ This is true!

B. $67 - x = 36$ This is true!

C. $x - 36 = 67$ This is NOT true!

D. $x + 36 = 67$ This is true!

23) Answer: D.

Even numbers always end with a digit 0, 2, 4, 6 or 8.

Therefore, numbers 48, 22, 70 are the only even numbers.

24) Answer: 85.

5 spaghettis with meatballs cost: 5 × $15 = $75

2 bowls of bean soup cost: 2 × $5 = $10

5 spaghettis with meatballs + 2 bowls of bean soup cost: $75 + $ 10 = $85

25) Answer: B.

$12 \times 55 = 660$

26) Answer: A.

1 hour = 60 minutes

2 hours = 2 × 60 minutes ⟹ 2hours = 120 minutes

27) Answer: C.

$32 \times 15 = 480$

28) Answer: 550.

We round the number up to the nearest ten if the last digit in the number is 5, 6, 7, 8, or 9.

We round the number down to the nearest ten if the last digit in the number is 1, 2, 3, or 4.

If the last digit is 0, then we do not have to do any rounding, because it is already rounded to the ten.

Therefore, rounded number of 547 to the nearest ten is 550.

29) Answer: A.

The table is divided into 100 equal parts. 72 parts of these 100 parts are shaded. It means $\frac{72}{100}$.

30) Answer: B.

Bryan city with 14,021 has the least population. Longview, Edinburg and Mission are other cities in order from least to greatest.

"End"